DR. SE DEVELOPED PROSTATE SIMPLIFIED

A simplified and treatment manual on how to cure developed prostate problems through Dr. Sebi diet

EMILY TOWNSEND

TABLE OF CONTENTS

CHAPTER ONE

INTRODUCTION

What food sources are useful for a developed prostate?

The prostate organ is a little, pecan formed organ that sits behind the bladder in men. During sexual action, the prostate organ helps produce semen, the supplement rich liquid that conveys the sperm during discharge.

As certain men get more seasoned, the prostate organ can become amplified, a condition known as harmless prostatic hyperplasia or BPH.

Dr. Sebi Diet and an expanded prostate

Strawberries, blueberries, raspberries, and blackberries are suggested as a feature of an augmented prostate eating routine.

The prostate organ is constrained by amazing chemicals known as the sex chemicals, including testosterone.

In the prostate organ, testosterone is changed over to another chemical called dihydrotestosterone (DHT). Undeniable degrees of DHT cause the cells in the prostate to augment.

Certain food sources and refreshments are known to affect prostate wellbeing as a result of their impacts on testosterone and different chemicals.

Exploration has tracked down that an eating routine fundamentally comprising of meat or dairy items can build the danger of prostate broadening and disease. This is particularly obvious if an individual doesn't fuse enough vegetables into their eating routine.

CHAPTER TWO

FOOD VARIETIES TO EAT

D r. Sebi diet wealthy in organic products, vegetables, and solid fats is thought to ensure the prostate.

Explicit food varieties known to help the prostate include:

Salmon:

Salmon is wealthy in solid fats that contain omega-3 unsaturated fats, which help forestall and diminish aggravation inside the body. Other cold-water fish, like sardines and trout, are likewise wealthy in these kinds of fats.

There are a lot of motivations to remember omega-3 unsaturated fats for your eating regimen. Omega-3s assist with bringing down terrible cholesterol and raise great cholesterol levels, lower hypertension, assist with weight reduction, and can diminish the danger of cardiovascular failure. In spite of the fact that specialists normally suggest eliminating creature fat for prostate wellbeing, an eating routine high in omega-3s can assist with boosting prostate wellbeing. Indeed, omega-3 unsaturated fats, found in food sources like lake trout and herring, may really assist with bringing down prostate malignant growth hazard.

Tomatoes:

Tomatoes are loaded with lycopene, a cancer prevention agent that might help prostate organ cells. This staple of late spring eating is without fat, sans sodium, and high in nutrients An and C. Watermelon is likewise a superb wellspring of lycopene, the cell reinforcement that gives entire food sources like tomatoes and watermelons their shading.

Examination proposes that lycopene might assist with bringing down prostate disease hazard. Lycopene can be found in food varieties like tomatoes, apricots, pink grapefruit, guava, and papaya. There are around 9 to 13 milligrams of lycopene in a cup and a portion of watermelon.

Berries:

Strawberries, blueberries, raspberries, and blackberries are amazing wellsprings of cancer prevention agents, which help to eliminate free extremists from the body. Free revolutionaries are the results of responses that happen inside the body and can cause harm and infection after some time.

Broccoli:

Broccoli and other cruciferous vegetables, including bok choy, cauliflower, Brussels fledglings, and cabbage, contain a compound known as sulforaphane. This is thought to target malignant growth cells and advance a solid prostate.

Nuts:

Nuts are plentiful in zinc, a minor element. Zinc is found in high fixations in the prostate and is thought to assist with adjusting testosterone and DHT. Other than nuts, shellfish and vegetables are additionally high in zinc.

Citrus:

Oranges, lemons, limes, and grapefruits are generally high in nutrient C, which might assist with ensuring the prostate organ.

Berries like strawberries, blackberries, and raspberries are high in nutrient C and cancer prevention agents. Cancer prevention agents assume a significant part in the body as they keep harm from free revolutionaries, particles that assault solid cells and can add to malignancy hazard. Nutrient C may likewise assist with facilitating harmless prostatic hyperplasia (BPH) indications by advancing pee and decreasing expanding.

Other incredible wellsprings of nutrient C incorporate citrus organic products, melon, spinach, broccoli, and mangos. For most grown-up men, 90 milligrams of nutrient C is suggested every day.

Onions and garlic:

One investigation discovered that men with BPH would in general eat less garlic and onions that men without BPH. More exploration is expected to affirm these outcomes, yet onions and garlic are restorative augmentations to most eating regimens.

CHAPTER THREE

FOOD VARIETIES TO STAY AWAY FROM

Caffeine ought to be stayed away from as a component of an eating routine for an augmented prostate.

A refreshing eating regimen for an augmented prostate is something beyond eating great food sources. It additionally implies staying away from different kinds of food varieties that are not useful for the prostate.

A few food varieties to stay away from include:

Red meat: Exploration proposes that going red sans meat might assist with working on prostate wellbeing. Truth be told, every day meat utilization is accepted to significantly increase the danger of prostate expansion.

Dairy: Comparably to meat, standard utilization of dairy has been connected to an expanded danger of BPH. Removing or decreasing margarine, cheddar, and milk might assist with diminishing BPH indications.

Caffeine: Caffeine might go about as a diuretic, which implies that it expands how a lot, how frequently, and how direly an individual needs to pee. Scaling back espresso, tea, pop, and chocolate might work on urinary manifestations of BPH.

Liquor: Liquor can likewise invigorate pee creation. Men with BPH might find that their indications are improved by surrendering liquor.

Sodium: A high salt admission might expand the urinary plot side effects related with BPH. Following a low-sodium diet by not adding salt to dinners and staying away from handled food varieties might be useful for certain men.

Dealing With an Expanded Prostate

Dietary changes can be very viable in dealing with a portion of the manifestations of BPH, yet other fundamental way of life changes can help also.

A few methodologies that might ease BPH side effects include:

- ✓ Overseeing pressure
- ✓ Stopping smoking
- ✓ Staying away from liquids in the evening to decrease evening pee
- ✓ Exhausting the bladder totally while peeing
- ✓ Doing pelvic floor works out

- ✓ Keeping away from meds that can demolish indications, like antihistamines, diuretics, and decongestants if conceivable
- ✓ Attempting bladder preparing works out
- ✓ Restricting liquid admission to 2 liters of fluids every day

Augmented Prostate Indications

The indications of an augmented prostate might incorporate trouble peeing and torment after discharge.

An extended prostate or BPH is genuinely normal. More than 14 million men in the US encountered BPH side effects in 2010.

Side effects of BPH include:

- ✓ Expanded urinary recurrence and earnestness
- ✓ Trouble beginning pee
- ✓ Feeble pee stream or spill toward the finish of pee
- ✓ Intruded on pee
- ✓ Continuous pee around evening time
- ✓ Incontinence
- ✓ torment after discharge
- ✓ Agonizing pee
- ✓ Urinary maintenance or powerlessness to pee

These manifestations happen when an augmented prostate organ hinders the urethra, the cylinder that runs between the bladder and outside of the body. This blockage can make it troublesome or even difficult to pass pee.

Treating BPH relies upon the seriousness of the indications. At times, just essential ways of life changes are required.

Notwithstanding, there are additionally meds or surgeries that can be powerful in diminishing the size of the prostate or the indications related with BPH.

CHAPTER FOUR

DIET ON WHEAT BREAD

11 stimulating options in contrast to wheat bread

Rye

Sourdough

Corn tortillas

Sans gluten

Sans gluten multiseed

Grown

Salad greens

Yams

Vegetables

Coconut flour

Cauliflower pizza

There are different reasons why an individual might wish to stay away from or eat less wheat bread. Luckily, there are numerous invigorating without wheat choices to browse.

Individuals who might wish to keep away from wheat-based bread include:

Those with celiac sickness, an immune system condition making stomach related manifestations in response eating food varieties containing gluten, for example, wheat-based items.

Those with different kinds of gluten-related issues.

The individuals who are following a low carb diet.

The people who don't care for the flavor of wheat bread.

The people who have settled on an individual decision to stay away from wheat bread for another explanation.

Numerous sans wheat bread options are accessible, permitting those after a decreased wheat or sans wheat diet to partake in their most loved sandwiches, wraps, toasts, and pizzas.

Choices to bread produced using wheat.

1. Rye bread

Rye bread is wealthy in fiber.

Rye bread is hazier, denser bread than wheat bread and is wealthy in fiber.

Experts:

Accessible in many stores and pastry shops

Generally easy to prepare at home

Cons:

More grounded and more mixed bag

not without gluten or appropriate for those with celiac sickness, non-celiac gluten-affectability or sensitivity, or other motivation to stay away from gluten

2. Sourdough bread

Individuals make sourdough bread from aged grains, making absorption simpler than numerous different breads.

While cooks use wheat in numerous sourdough breads, individuals can likewise discover or prepare sourdough bread from rye or without gluten flour.

Experts:

Longer aging interaction might make supplements more accessible and help processing

Sans gluten flour can be utilized when making sans gluten sourdough bread

Individuals can prepare it at home

Contains probiotics, which support solid gut microorganisms

Cons:

Have a harsh and more mixed bags

Sweet garnishes, like jam or nectar, may not work with the sharp taste

Not everything is sans gluten, and supermarkets will in general stock wheat-based sourdough bread

3. Corn tortillas

Corn tortillas will be tortillas delivered from corn, making them an incredible sans gluten, high-fiber alternative. Individuals use them for tacos and other Mexican dishes, yet additionally as wraps and pizza bases.

Experts:

Sans gluten

Generally accessible

Simple to discover when eating out

Simple to make at home

Lower carbs and calories than wheat choices

Cons:

Look and feel altogether different to wheat bread

Not reasonable for individuals with corn prejudice or sensitivity

4. Sans gluten bread

A few stores sell numerous assortments of sans gluten bread.

Without gluten bread is the easiest method to stay away from wheat and gluten.

Experts:

Both without gluten bread and without gluten flour are promptly accessible

Simple to make at home

Many sorts, brands, and formula alternatives to browse

Cons:

Sans gluten bread tastes distinctive to wheat bread

Needs a bigger number of fixings than wheat bread

5. Without gluten multiseed bread

Multiseed bread is a thick bread containing a wide range of seeds.

Experts:

Without gluten

Seeds are a decent wellspring of protein and sound fats

Easy to make

Cons:

Frequently not accessible when eating out or at stores

Normally, a denser bread than wheat bread.

6. Grown bread

Individuals cause grew bread from grains they to have permitted to grow or grow. Grown grains can include:

Wheat

Millet

Spelt

Grain

Soybeans

Lentils

There are sans gluten and without wheat grew bread alternatives that do exclude any wheat or gluten-containing grains.

Experts:

Grown grains might make the bread simpler to process

Sans gluten assortments are accessible

Regularly accessible at general stores

Individuals can make it at home

Cons:

Many grew breads contain wheat and gluten so make certain to peruse the marks

Less accessible when eating out

More hard to make than some different sorts of bread

7. Lettuce and salad greens

Large mixed greens, like lettuce, collard greens, and kale can be an incredible replacement for wraps and bread. Individuals can simply top or fill huge leaves with any fixings, including veggies, cheddar, meat, avocados, and hummus. Then, at that point they just need to move the leaves up, crease them, or eat them level.

Experts:

High in supplements and low in calories

Sans gluten

Low in carbs

Promptly accessible

Cons:

Try not to suggest a flavor like bread

Can be more chaotic than bread

8. Yams

Yams are a supplement rich choice to bread.

Yam cuts can be a great substitute for bread. They can be utilized with any fixings and can even be toasted.

Experts:

Wealthy in supplements and fiber

Without gluten

Delicious and inventive

Cons:

Try not to suggest a flavor like bread

9. Vegetables

A few vegetables make a great substitute for bread. Eggplants, huge mushrooms, and chime peppers can be utilized rather than buns and cut bread. Cucumbers and carrots are astounding for plunging rather than breadsticks and wheat wafers.

Experts:

Wealthy in supplements and fiber

Low in calories

Without gluten

Lower in carbs

Delicious and innovative

Cons:

Try not to suggest a flavor like bread

10. Coconut flour and squash flatbread

Making flatbread with coconut flour and butternut squash, yams, or pumpkin is an innovative and delicious flatbread option in contrast to wheat bread.

Experts:

Sans gluten

Easy to make

Cons:

Not accessible at stores

11. Cauliflower pizza covering

Cauliflower pizza covering has become well known lately. Individuals utilize ground cauliflowers, eggs, cheddar, and flavors when making these bases.

Experts:

Without gluten

Simple to make

Low-carb

Some supermarkets sell frozen cauliflower pizza bases

Cons:

Tastes distinctive to normal pizza outside

Incorporates eggs and dairy so unacceptable for veggie lovers or those with dairy or eggs bigotries or sensitivities

CHAPTER FIVE

DR. SEBI DIET FOR VEGGIE LOVER

What to think about veggie lover dinner arranging.

Many individuals follow a vegetarian diet, which includes eating plant-based food varieties and barring every creature item, like meat, dairy, and eggs. In spite of the fact that it can at first be hard to get the right equilibrium of supplements, setting up a feast intend to follow the eating regimen effectively can assist individuals with staying away from inadequacies.

When beginning a vegetarian diet, it could be troublesome at first to recognize proper substitutes for creature items and accomplish the right dietary profile. Numerous things inside a veggie lover diet can be profoundly nutritious and further develop parts of wellbeing. Nonetheless, individuals likewise need to see how to get certain supplements, like iron, calcium, and nutrient B12, which it can at times be trying to incorporate enough of in a vegetarian diet.

In this book, we talk about the advantages and dangers of veganism and give some veggie lover feast ideas to breakfast, lunch, and supper.

What is veganism?

Veganism commonly includes the avoidance of creature items, like meat, poultry, and fish, just as creature side-effects, including eggs, nectar, and dairy. All things considered, individuals burn-through plant-based food varieties, like vegetables, natural products, nuts, seeds, vegetables, and soy. Many individuals who follow a vegetarian diet likewise stay away from all types of creature items, including certain garments, and items that include creature testing.

The Foundation of Nourishment and Dietetics expresses that vegetarian dietary examples can be different, nutritious, and supportive for the avoidance and the executives of some constant conditions.

Advantages

Individuals might pick a veggie lover way of life for an assortment of reasons. For instance, certain individuals might embrace veggie lover dietary examples for individual, strict, ecological, or wellbeing reasons.

Dodges pitilessness to animals

Eating a vegetarian diet utilizing Dr. Sebi diet technique implies not devouring any meat or creature results. Not eating creature items can assist with lessening the interest, conceivably diminishing the quantity of creatures that individuals breed and kill for food. A large number of the individuals who follow a vegetarian diet refer to staying away from creature brutality as one of the fundamental purposes behind their decision.

Weight reduction

A nutritious veggie lover diet will incorporate a wide assortment of vegetables, which are normally low in calories. Albeit the quantity of calories changes fundamentally among various vegetarian dinners, a few examinations show a connection between eating a veggie lover diet and weight reduction.

A little 2015 review affecting 50 individuals who were overweight looked at the impacts of an omnivorous eating routine, a semi-veggie lover diet, a veggie lover diet, and a vegetarian diet on weight reduction. Individuals who ate a veggie lover diet revealed more weight reduction than different gatherings.

Diminished danger of coronary illness

A plant-based eating regimen, for example, a veggie lover diet, may lessen the danger of coronary illness. Exploration in Progress in Cardiovascular Sicknesses Believed Source demonstrates that heart-solid way of life decisions might diminish the danger of a coronary episode by about 80%.

Scientists have related plant-based eating regimens with a 40% decrease in cardiovascular illness passings and the danger of coronary course infection. Following a plant-based eating routine might bring about diminished cholesterol and circulatory strain, just as a diminished danger of creating type 2 diabetes.

Staple things that individuals may wish to consider adding to a veggie lover shopping rundown could include:

Grains: Models incorporate rice, quinoa, and oats.

Natural products: Individuals can browse a wide reach, including peaches, melons, berries, apples, and avocados.

Vegetables: Great choices incorporate dim salad greens, cauliflower, peppers, and yams.

Bundled: Saltines, cereal, and soups are valuable storeroom staples.

Flavorings: Balsamic vinegar, escapades, olive oil, pepper, turmeric, and different spices, flavors, and dressings can make suppers more flavorsome.

Protein sources

As a vegetarian diet does exclude meat, eat food sources that contain protein. Great wellsprings of protein on a vegetarian diet include:

Tofu

Beans

Vegetables

Nuts

Almond margarine

Chickpeas

Lentils

Dairy and egg options

Options in contrast to dairy items might include:

Canned coconut milk

Veggie lover egg substitutes

Iron sources

Some veggie lover wellsprings of iron might include:

Chickpeas

Tofu

Cashew nuts

Chia seeds

Hemp seeds

Braced breakfast oats

Calcium sources

Vegetarian wellsprings of calcium include:

Strengthened tofu

Strengthened plant milk

Sustained yogurt choices

Sustained bread

Kale

Watercress

Okra

Almonds

Nutrient B12 sources

Some vegetarian items containing nutrient B12 include:

Nutrient B12 supplements

Braced plant milks

Braced oats

Nourishing yeast

Tempeh

Nori ocean growth

Chlorella

Spirulina

CHAPTER SIX

DR. SEBI DIET FEAST PLAN MODEL

Different cookbooks and sites offer an enormous assortment of supper thoughts for individuals who follow a vegetarian diet. While building a vegetarian supper plan, individuals ought to guarantee that they are getting adequate sustenance.

The following is an illustration of a potential 3-day veggie lover feast plan:

Breakfast	Lunch	Dinner	Snack
1 cup	black	tofu	hum

nondairy yogurt alternative topped with a quarter cup of strawberries and almonds	bean or soy burger with sliced tomatoes and baby spinach on a vegan bread roll	stir fry with 1 cup each of tofu, red and green peppers, and broccoli	mus with carrot and celery sticks
two slices of Ezekiel toast topped with a half cup of mashed	grain bowl with 1 cup of brown rice and 1	stuffed peppers with quinoa, onion, and	1 cup of mixed berries with a quart

avocado	cup of mixed carrots, edamame, peppers, and cherry tomatoes	tomato	er cup of walnuts
peanut butter banana oatmeal with a quarter cup of cooked rolled	2 cups of mixed salad greens with oil and vinegar, a	two corn tortillas with sauteed portobello mushr	1 cup of roasted edamame and chickpeas

oats, a half cup of sliced banana, a quarter cup of peanut butter, and soy or almond milk

quarte r cup of sunflo wer seeds, and 1 cup of mixed red pepper, carrot, cucum ber, and tomato

oom, onion, and cabbag e

Dangers and contemplations

There are additionally some likely dangers to following a veggie lover diet. Realizing the dangers assists a person with changing their eating routine and incorporate or avoid certain food sources for better generally speaking nourishment. Potential dangers might include:

Lacking protein: Individuals following certain veggie lover diets might battle to incorporate sufficient protein.

Supplement insufficiencies: Iron and some different supplements, for example, nutrient B12, are to a great extent in creature items.

Restricted food decisions eating out: Not all eateries have a vegetarian menu, which might make eating out testing.

With some arranging and thought, an individual might keep away from the dangers. They ought to think about the accompanying:

Recall key supplements: To keep away from dietary lacks, it is fundamental to eat food varieties containing nutrient B12, for example, braced oats and plant milks, and a lot of protein-rich food sources, like tofu, nuts, and beans.

Watch calories: Not all veggie lover food varieties are low in sugar or calories. For instance, veggie lover snacks, like treats, may have a high sugar content. Nuts and seeds are nutritious yet in addition high in calories, so individuals might wish to restrict their part estimates.

Eat an assortment of food sources: A veggie lover diet contains a ton of vegetables and organic products. Mixing it up of meat and dairy substitutes can assist a person with keeping an even eating routine.

Any individual who has specific worries about their eating routine or is uncertain how to make a reasonable dinner plan might wish to work with a certificd dietitian.

What to think about food sources that keep you conscious

Caffeine

Liquor

Zesty food sources

Sweet food varieties

Greasy food sources

Handled food sources

Caffeine

Many individuals devour caffeine, for instance, as espresso, to assist them with getting up in the first part of the day. Caffeine is likewise present in chocolate, tea, caffeinated beverages, and pop, like cola. Also, the substance expands alertness and feelings of excitement. A few people are additionally more touchy to caffeine's belongings because of hereditary contrasts, with more established grown-ups being more inclined than more youthful grown-ups.

Liquor

In spite of the fact that liquor is a depressant, it doesn't advance soothing rest. Albeit certain individuals might nod off rapidly in the wake of devouring liquor, they frequently end up getting up sooner than expected and attempting to return to rest.

Liquor likewise meddles with the circadian mood, demolishing rest quality. It can likewise adversely influence rest apnea.

Zesty food sources

Hot food sources may adversely influence rest severally. They can cause acid reflux, indigestion, and acid reflux, making it feel off kilter to rests. Furthermore, heartburn can demolish rest apnea. These food varieties likewise raise internal heat level, making it hard to get adequately cool to nod off serenely.

The capacity to bear heat from bean stew peppers, inside in numerous hot food sources, and its impacts on the body, fluctuates from one person to another. For those individuals who track down that devouring hot food varieties contrarily influences rest, it could be ideal to try not to eat them some time before sleep time.

Sweet and high glycemic file food varieties

Food varieties that cause a spike in glucose, like white rice, potatoes, candy, and other sweet food varieties, are called high glycemic food varieties.

Burning-through these food sources makes glucose rise quickly, bringing about the arrival of insulin, which influences tryptophan and serotonin levels. There is additionally an intricate collaboration of insulin with adrenalin, cortisol, glucagon, and development chemical, all of which can adversely affect rest.

Greasy food sources

Devouring high fat substance food varieties, like greasy meats and treats, may likewise upset rest. The body's absorption normally eases back when an individual rests. Greasy food sources will make the stomach feel full and may cause it hard for people to feel good.

They can likewise cause heartburn and indigestion, which are additionally prone to bring about helpless rest quality.

Prepared food varieties

Profoundly prepared food varieties incorporate inexpensive food and prepackaged food sources. While advantageous, these food varieties contain large numbers of the dietary parts above, including sugars and fats, which adversely sway rest.

THE END